Y✿GA

7 Minutes a Day
7 Days a Week

Dear Carol,

We can do this

together

Love

Jack o "R"

2/22/18

8/22/18

YOGA

7 Minutes a Day
7 Days a Week

A Gentle Daily Practice
for Strength, Clarity, and Calm

GERTRUD HIRSCHI

Conari Press

First English language edition 2017
by Conari Press, an imprint of
Red Wheel/Weiser, LLC
With offices at:
65 Parker Street, Suite 7
Newburyport, MA 01950
www.redwheelweiser.com

ISBN: 978-1-57324-697-2
Library of Congress Cataloging-in-Publication Data available upon request.

Cover design by Jim Warner
Photos of yoga exercises by Manuel Vargas Lépiz
Mudras illustrations by Hermann Betken (reprinted by kind permission of
Königsfurt-Urania Verlages)
All interior decorative photography © Bigstock.com or © Fotofolia.com and may not be
reproduced without permission.

Printed in Canada
MAR
10 9 8 7 6 5 4 3 2 1

Disclaimer: The advice published in this book has been carefully prepared and reviewed,
and is presented without guarantee of outcome. The author and publisher assume
no liability for personal injury; a medical professional should be consulted before
rigorous practice.

CONTENTS

The path leads from unattainable to attainable.

AN INTRODUCTION TO THE PRACTICE

*T*wenty years ago I created a small booklet in which I briefly described the qualities that I associate with each day of the week, and I provided suggestions for corresponding yoga exercises and a meditation guide for each day. I received tremendous positive feedback, and this current book expands upon that approach, providing a yoga exercise program that you can practice seven minutes a day, seven days a week, for strength, clarity, and calm.

It doesn't matter how young or old you are, the yoga exercises presented here are simple and can be followed no matter what your limitation may be. Your body will thank you with more energy, flexibility, and positive emotion.

Regular meditation is also part of a yoga regimen. Meditation connects the human consciousness with the universe. Used in conjunction with these daily yoga practices, meditation provides a source of security, trust, serenity, ease, inner peace, and freedom.

For many years I have asked myself, what makes people happy and what makes their lives feel fulfilled? It became clear to me that in our lives nothing superhuman is expected of us. Satisfied, successful, and happy people all have clear plans for their lives and are always setting new goals—simple goals, complex goals, but goals nonetheless. When they reach one goal, they move on to the next, step by step. Happy people are patient, flexible, committed, and steadfast. They also pay close attention to their circumstances, to the *here and now*.

Most of all, happy people are able to let go and simply trust in something larger than themselves. May this book be a steady guide for you, and may the exercises benefit you and bring you joy.

—Gertrud Hirschi

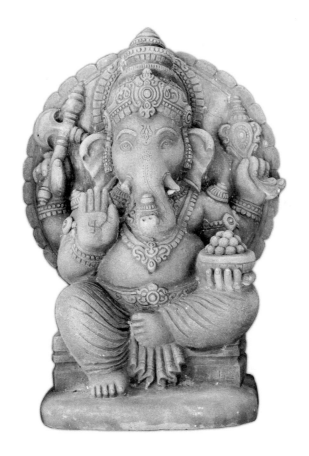

Ganesh is the Deity of the spring, of new beginnings, and of
success. May he bring you prosperity and joy.

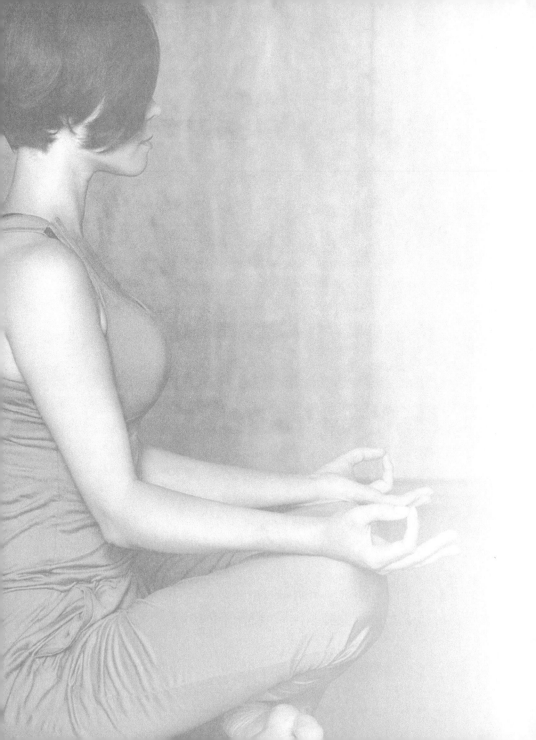

MEDITATIONS, MANTRAS, AND MUDRAS

*L*ife always presents us with new obstacles and challenges. Yoga can't protect us from them, but, with a yoga-minded lifestyle, we can cope with and overcome them. Regular and well-practiced meditation, mantras, and mudras are crucial to this yoga regimen; we turn inward through our breathing, which turns us toward mindfulness. Each of the seven yoga sequences in this book will include meditation, mantras, and mudras.

Meditation

Meditation is about resting, contemplating, gathering insight and foresight, all of which can considerably alleviate the stress in our lives and transform us into level-headed people who not only can help ourselves but also help those in need.

The gifts of the yoga sequences in this book are many; among them are mental and emotional strength, spiritual clarity, and a higher awareness. These benefits can then be applied to our meditations to develop life strategies for creating and achieving our life goals or simply to create a beautiful moment of peace when we need it.

Mantras

If we see meditation as the structure, then the mantras are the colors we use to paint. They improve our concentration, reinforce our resolve, and focus our intention. The recitations of the mantras in this book might seem easy to understand on their face, but this can be misleading because the content of the mantra can sound like something we simply *want* or *would like* to be. Mantras repeated without intent and awareness can make us feel like we are only trying to fool ourselves.

Here is an example of this: Let us say you are deeply unhappy and you boldly declare: *I am happy and content.* Does that really work? Should you just tell yourself that until you believe the lie? Of course, a mantra of this sort is not our *intention.* I have recently learned an interesting method to remedy this exact issue. I learned it from the practitioner Siranus Sven von Staden; he recommends that you should recite the mantra as a question and then reply with your own answer, which your mind will readily produce on its own. The transformed mantra might now sound like: *Why am I happy*

*and content? Because I am healthy . . . because I have a family
. . . because I live in this country . . .*

In this way, we can connect our consciousness with the positive and not with deficiency, and thus we can initiate the fulfillment of our mantra. This is what is meant by intention.

Mudras

Mudras are spiritual and specific hand gestures. In yoga, mudras are often used in conjunction with breathing to stimulate the flow of *prana*—the life force—in the body. In this book, the recommended mudras provided along with the yoga sequences give the exercise a foundation and wake the energy that is needed for development. All of our energy paths are connected to corresponding emotions and thought structures. Is the energy weak? Or blocked? Or is it activated and strong?

The mudras are easy to practice. Keep your hands loose and without any pressure in your fingers. There is nothing you can do wrong!

I like to recommend beginning with a thorough hand massage, by palpating and rubbing each hand. Lace your fingers together, and then let them slide apart. This will activate the ten energy meridians that extend along the sides of the fingers.

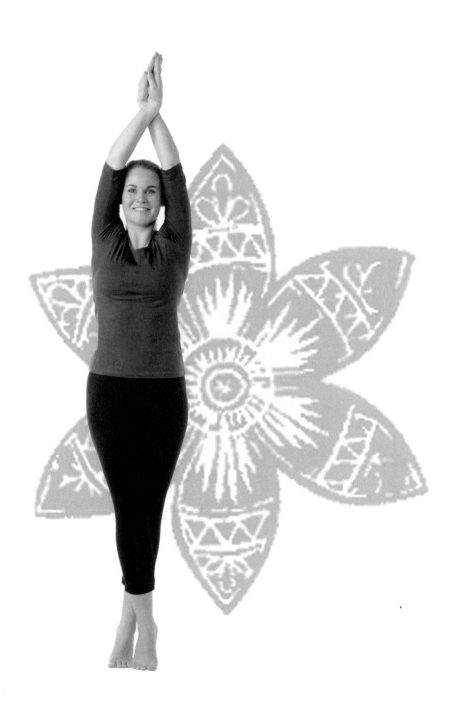

ABOUT
THE YOGA POSTURES

*W*hile compiling the yoga routines for this book, I sought to include postures and movements that would provide a great deal of benefit in seven simple exercises, all of which are understandable and manageable for everyone.

If I haven't included special instructions for breathing, this means that you should simply let your breath flow effortlessly.

The specified number of repetitions or the number of breaths or the length of time to hold the position can be changed at your discretion. As you become more accustomed to the movements and to your own body, you will discover what is right for you. Less can often be more.

You will notice that there are no extremely exacting instructions for each yoga pose. Correct form is, of course, very important. However, this is a book for beginners as well as experienced practitioners, for young and old alike. Some postures are more difficult than others; many people may not be able to fully extend their arms such as indicated in Chest Expander or Bird in the Nest, and many people will find the Candle Pose difficult.

In all cases, read the instructions and put yourself in the position as it is pictured, to the best of your ability. Your form does not have to be perfect! Experienced yoga practitioners will find these poses familiar. If you are a beginner, you will find the more you practice, the stronger and more limber you will become. What *is* important is reaping the physical, emotional, and spiritual benefits from each pose, and these poses have been specifically chosen with that in mind.

The closing resting position

Each daily sequence closes with the resting position. This is very important. After each exercise series, you should make yourself comfortable in the resting position (put a cushion under your knees if you like) and make sure you are warm. It is important that you not let your thoughts wander or slip into a negative direction. Instead, consciously connect your thoughts to something positive or think of a goal you would like to achieve. Or recite the suggested mantra that I have included.

The resting position reinforces the outcome of the yoga exercises on all levels in a short amount of time.

Please be aware of the following precautions:

❊ Don't begin your exercise after a heavy meal.

❊ These exercises were created for people in good health. Do not practice the daily routine if you are ill or have a medical condition, have any kind of back pain or other injury, have unstable blood pressure, or have recently had any surgery.

Do the physical movements correctly

Read the instructions for the daily exercises prior to practicing them. This will allow you to make the most out of your few minutes a day.

✳ Collect yourself before you begin the practice.

✳ Do some warm-up exercises until you are relaxed, loose, and feel warm.

✳ Always inhale and exhale through your nose.

✳ When you hold a pose, keep your breathing effortless and consistent.

✳ Make all movements flow with consciousness; move smoothly and slowly, keeping in sync with your breathing.

✳ For asymmetrical positions, hold each side for an equal number of breaths.

✳ Remain in the resting position for at least seven minutes after the exercises. Allow plenty of time to enjoy the relaxation. Resting will multiply the effects of the entire routine.

EVERY DAY
IS SPECIAL

*D*ecide that every day is a new beginning, and align yourself with the new
possibilities each day can bring.

Leave the past and future where
they are and enjoy the magic of the
moment—the here and now. Keep your evenings free of retrospection and say thank you for all the good the day has brought
you.

The exercises for each individual day follow a harmonious
theme. On one hand, each daily routine is separate; however,
each daily sequence is balanced with all the others to make a
whole. Each yoga sequence focuses on a specific body area and
health benefit that resonates with the energy of that particular
day. For example, Sunday holds the energy of the sun, and the
sun represents fire and life-giving energy. Therefore on Sunday
the yoga exercises are designed to strengthen your heart—your
life giving organ—and harmonize your circulatory system.
Monday, the day of the moon, represents your emotions and

the fluid systems of your body—and so on through the seven days of the week.

At the end of the week you will find that you have done something beneficial for each area of your body. And keep in mind that you can certainly follow the same daily routine over several days if there is some specific body system you want to work on.

$\mathcal{S}unday$

DAY OF THE SUN

ven the ancients dedicated the first day of the week to the sun. For millennia the sun has been a symbol of the Divine.

Sunday represents a new day in which a new beginning is hiding, lying in wait. Everything that germinates and grows has its source in peace and serenity. Think of a child in the womb or the butterfly in its cocoon, the seeds deep in the earth, or flowers in the bulbs—everything that grows and unfolds first has its start in the dark and concealed. Therefore, the sun is connected to birth and growth. The sun awakens life, and life is attracted to the light.

The sun affects everything in nature, including our physical body, our emotions, and our spiritual being. Many of us feel a sense of tranquility on a warm summer afternoon, especially in our moods and thinking. The sun can make you so relaxed that you may not want to put the effort into concentration or take on heavy emotions. Following such a time of relaxation, there is a new sense of creative power, new ideas, and vigor. In many cultures and religions, Sunday was a mandated day of rest. Perhaps many of our modern-day stresses could be reduced if we reinstated Sunday as a rest day. You don't have to make it religious; simply use the day to laze about to your heart's content.

It is best to leave a little time on Sunday to contemplate your new beginning, or even better, to write down your ideas and create a plan for the week. This will help you implement those ideas over the coming days.

On a physical level, Sunday corresponds to the circulatory system. Chinese healers are known to consider circulation an element of fire, which therefore indicates the sun. A weakened heart often causes internal strife, ill-health, and creates obstacles for creating joy, empathy, and love. Problems with your heart will influence your entire personality. When you don't have your heart in shape, all sorts of difficulties will compound in your life. Stress, one of the greatest factors in heart-related disease, is often part of our weekday marathon of duties at home, school, and work, and there is often little we can do to avoid stressors during the week. But what about Sundays?

It is imperative that you regularly make time—and specifically on Sunday—for a conscious pause. Push all obligations away and indulge in relaxation. Try, with the best of intentions, to enjoy each moment of awareness. This will allow you to become a sun-oriented person: generous, tolerant, and sympathetic. Construct every Sunday to be something special for you, following this motto: *Relax and do something beautiful.*

Exercise routine for the heart

The sun corresponds to the heart, circulation, and oxygen balance. Tension can make its way in behind the sternum and constrain or even block passages that nourish the heart. When the energy of the heart is weakened or restricted, the output of the heart is reduced. People who have suffered from cardiac issues will tend to fall into depression or find it difficult to find joy, compassion, and love. Therefore, we should make the point clear: *bring the sun into the heart.*

The first three Sunday exercises—Windmill, Arm Rotator, and Chest Twist—release tension in the chest area through compression and stretching. The Blade activates the energy meridian that is known as the Protector of the Heart. The mudra in Oak soothingly stimulates the entire chest. St. Andrew's Cross and Chest Expander invigorate your circulation.

Tips for throughout the day

❋ It doesn't matter if you are standing, sitting, or lying down; open your arms like you want to hug the world and briefly enjoy the moment, the feeling of vastness, freedom, and weightlessness.

❋ Grasp your pinky finger with four fingers of the opposite hand, this activates the meridians known as the Protector and Master Nourisher of the heart.

1. Windmill

✳ Stand in a relaxed position: one arm extended in front and the other reaching behind.

✳ Now move like the windmill, slowly and rhythmically moving your arms in circles, with one arm going up while the other is simultaneously going down.

✳ The same motion should be repeated with arms moving in the opposite direction.

✳ After six rotations in each direction, end by raising up both arms until your upper arms touch your ears, and then lower them.

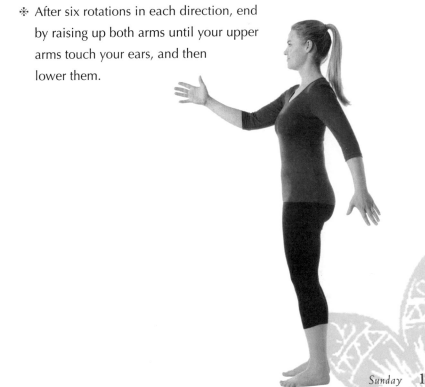

2. Arm Rotator

❉ Stand upright with hands placed on top of your head, fingers interlaced and palms up.

❉ Inhale and stretch your arms upward.

❉ Hold your breath as you bend your torso to the right and then to the left.

    ❉ Exhale slowly as you return to the upright position; slowly lower your hands to a resting position on your head.

    ❉ Repeat four times.

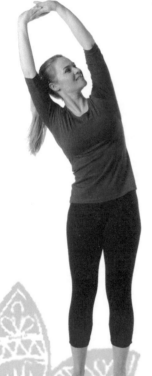

3. Chest Twist

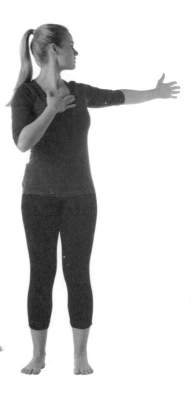

* Stand with your feet shoulder-width apart with your right hand on your chest.

* Inhale and raise your left arm to shoulder height.

* Exhale and slowly sweep your left arm across your body to the opposite side.

* Repeat four times.

* Change the hand positions and repeat four times.

4. Blade

* Stand with your fingertips pressed on your chest, head bowed, and knees slightly bent.

* Inhale and throw your head back and your arms behind your torso as you straighten your legs.

* Exhale and come back to the original position.

* Repeat six times.

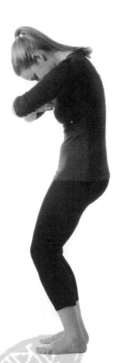
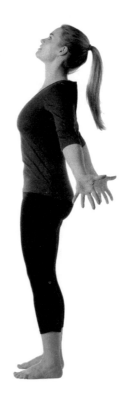

5. Oak

* ❊ Stand on your right foot with the left foot pressed against your right leg, the left heel touching the side of the right knee.

* ❊ Hands are pressed together, with thumbs pressing against the center of the chest. Concentrate on your heart and hold the position for fifteen breaths, while silently saying:

Thoughtfulness and peace
should fill my heart

* ❊ Repeat standing on the opposite foot.

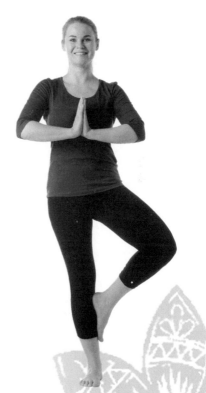

6. St. Andrew's Cross

�֍ Stand on the balls of your feet with your arms open
and stretched toward the sun—this opens up your inner
strength. Hold the position for ten to twenty breaths,
repeating silently:

I am grateful to be filled with this light, warmth, and joy.

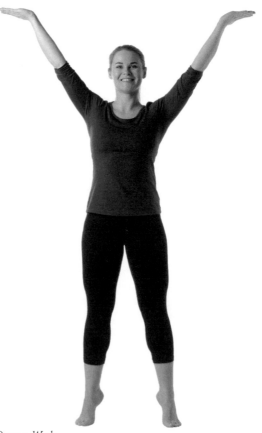

7. Chest Expander

✳ Standing upright, put your arms behind your body with hands together and fingers interlaced.

✳ Stretch your arms out and squeeze your shoulder blades together as you lean forward, bringing your torso toward your thighs.

✳ Stay in this crouched position for fifteen breaths and then return to the standing position.

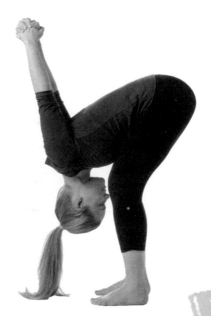

Closing Resting Position

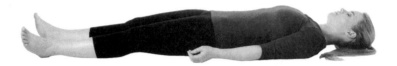

*The sun shall invigorate my body, bring light
to my spirit, and warm my soul.*

Meditation

Just as the sun provides energy for each plant to open its blooms, it can also open us to the universal consciousness and its gifts. A breathtaking opened blossom is a wonder of nature. The following meditation can bring joy, openness, and light into your life.

- Sit comfortably with a straightened spine or in your chosen meditation position. Now, take six deep breaths. With each exhale, direct your thoughts to the warmth in the breath as it goes out; let all tension go—in your face, shoulders, arms, chest, back, pelvis, and legs.
- Picture in your mind's eye: You are sitting with the sun's rays warming you. On your head is an opened flower. Breathe in and take in the flowing light. Breathe out letting go of negativity and feeling your heart open.
- Finish the meditation being thankful for the universal consciousness in every second of your life.

Mantra

I open myself to the Divine joy.
May it fill my heart as I go into the world.

Mudra

- Your hands are open like unfurled blossoms, resting on your thighs.
- This will activate your Heart meridian and hand chakras.

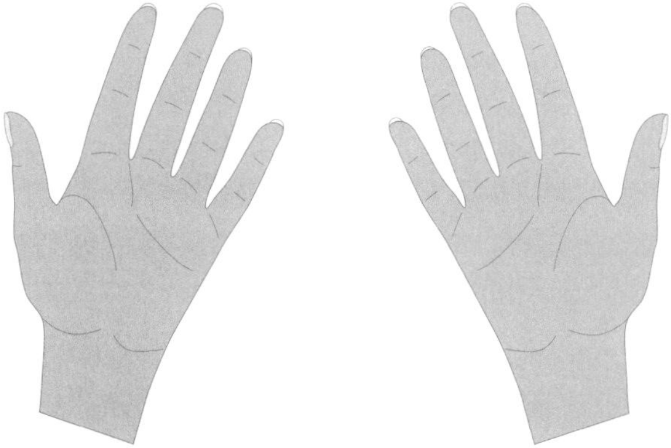

Monday

DAY OF THE MOON

Monday is moon day. This day follows Sunday because it, like the moon, doesn't send out its own light, but rather reflects the sun—Monday doesn't assert much clarity. You often hear of people talking about the "Monday blues." But if you are fully awake on Mondays, you will find a deeper symbolism for the day. The moon influences many things, and there is nothing on earth that isn't directly or indirectly influenced by the moon. It moves the oceans, regulates how crops and plants grow, changes animal behavior, affects the menstrual cycle, and alters the mood and spirit of people. The moon speaks to the deepest layers of our spirit. Traumas from our early childhood or hidden feelings can be brought back to our attention by the position of the moon. During a full moon, people tend to have more dreams through which the subconscious exposes troublesome patterns. These then can be corrected or put to rest.

The moon corresponds to the feminine in every person. Several aspects of the feminine are conformity, suffering in silence, as well as patience and feeling the power to create serenity.

Melancholy and petulance are also influenced by the moon. Usually, a bad mood can be changed or turned around if you are willing to admit something in earnest or if you can distance yourself from it as much as possible. "I am in a foul mood, but I won't let it ruin my day!"

Mondays are suited for indulging in memories simply because it is helpful to to look back at experiences and be able to draw out a lesson from them. How often do we use Mondays to ruminate on annoying or troublesome things from the weekend? Yet we tend to fall back into the same patterns, never having fully analyzed the circumstances. You meet up with people you don't really like or get caught up in doing things that you really don't want to do, or you forget to do something really important . . . the list goes on and on. Mondays should be for planning and retrospection—making and creating new patterns for the coming week that will make you happy.

Mondays are suited for cathartic processes with water. Make a cleansing ritual for this time. Do this with forgiveness in mind, and forgive yourself whenever you can as healing old wounds will free you from the past. Some of us might find it difficult to simply forgive. In this case, ask the Divine for help.

You can also use Monday to quietly enter a nicer memory or a sweet melancholy as you wait for Tuesday, at which time everything will look completely different.

Exercise routine for the pelvic area

The moon works on the body's water balance system: lymph system, spleen, bladder, and kidneys. The following yoga routine allows the lymph nodes and surrounding areas to stretch and be pressed, allowing for increased circulation and relaxation in the pelvic area. There is a lot of tension hidden in the pelvic region and it blocks intestinal flow, causing discomfort and pain during menstruation. In the first movement, Bamboo, the abdominal area is stretched and compressed; in Butterfly the pelvic floor and the sex organs are unblocked. Side Arch, Broth Mixer, and Swivel Seat tighten and release the same areas. In Crocodile all tension is again released. Candle closes the sequence and optimizes circulation in the pelvic area.

Tips for throughout the day

❋ If you read or watch TV at night, try sitting in the Butterfly position. In this position you can hold your feet or gently sit on them.

❋ Occasionally wrap the fingers of one hand around the pinky finger (representing the small intestine) of the other hand or around the pointer finger (for the large intestine).

1. Bamboo

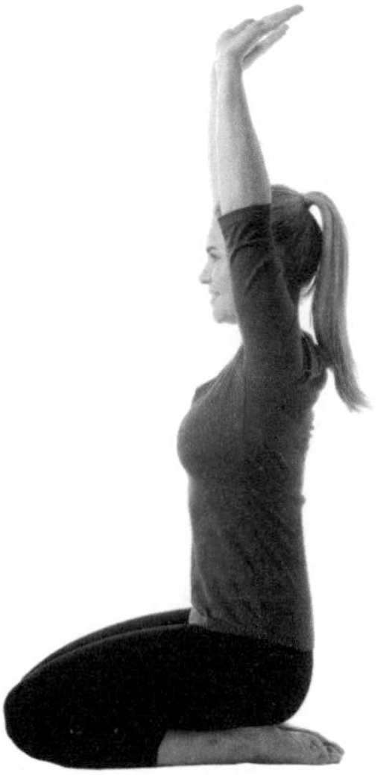

- ❈ Sit on your heels.
- ❈ As you inhale slowly, reach your arms up, palms facing upward.
- ❈ Hold your breath as you stretch your torso upward.
- ❈ Exhale and slowly bend forward.
- ❈ Breathe in as you return to an upright position.
- ❈ Hold your breath as you reach behind you and place your palms on the ground behind your raised buttocks.

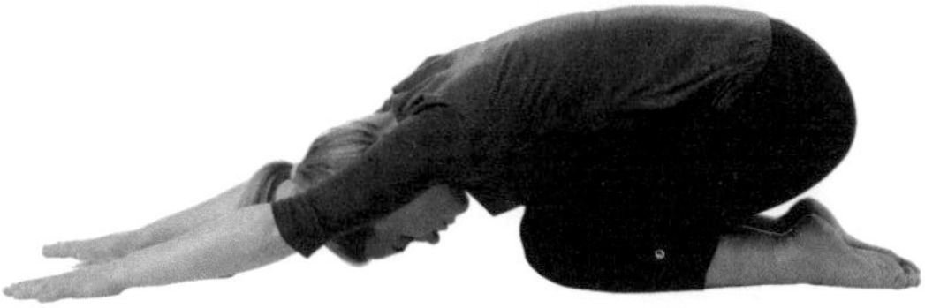

- ❈ Exhale as you return to the seated position.
- ❈ Repeat six times.

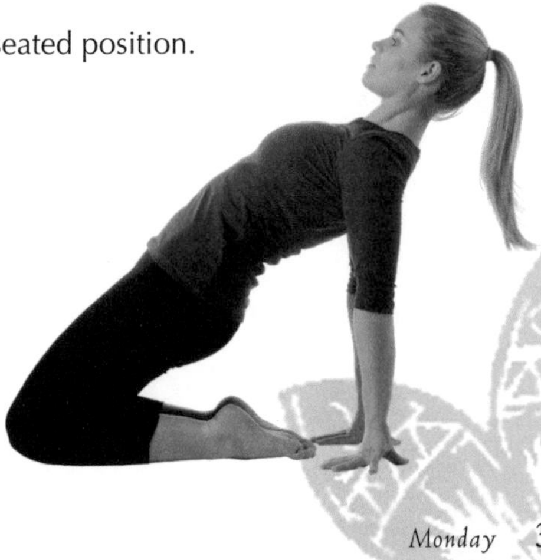

2. Butterfly

- ✻ Sitting with your knees pointed outward and the soles of the feet pressed together, gently move your knees up and down to send vibrations to the pelvis.
- ✻ Relax and let a sense of well-being preside over you.

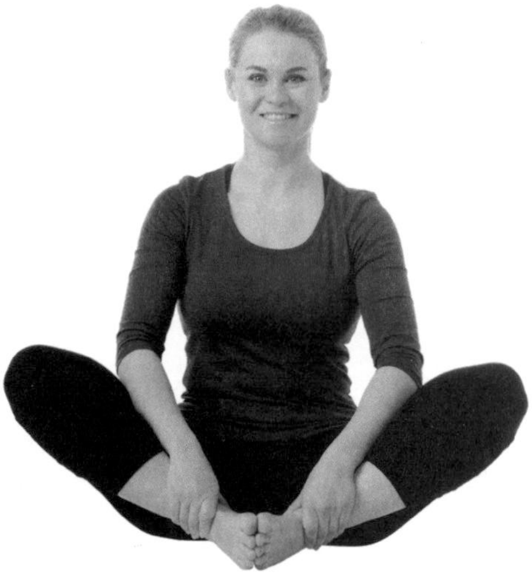

3. Side Arch

❊ Inhale and press your right hand on the ground and stretch your left arm upward, palm facing you.

❊ Hold your breath and stretch your left side by arching to the right.

❊ Exhale as you let your arm return to your lap.

❊ Repeat on each side four times.

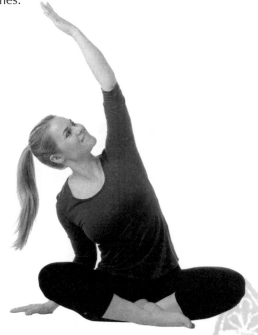

4. Broth Mixer (Witch's Cauldron)

✳ In front of you is a large cauldron on a fire. You are stirring the magical soup clockwise and counterclockwise, six times in each direction.

✳ Be careful, the edge is hot and can burn you, so stretch out far!

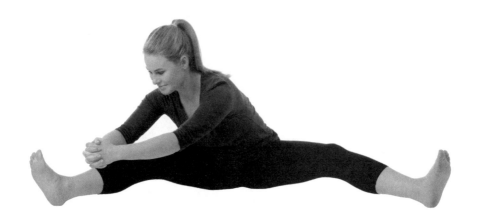

5. Swivel Seat

❋ Press your right leg with bended knee against your body; feel the heat that is generated.

❋ Turn your torso to the left and extend your left arm out at shoulder height. Look at your left hand.

❋ Take ten deep breaths as you hold this position.

❋ Repeat with the other leg.

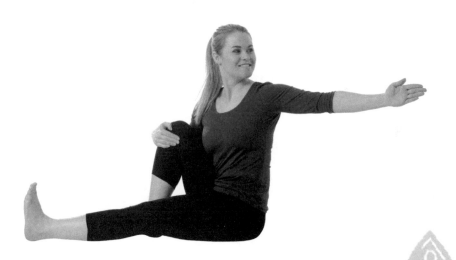

6. Crocodile 1

✢ Lay on your back with legs bent and together, feet pressed flat to the ground, and fingers pressed on the top of the skull.

✢ Breathe out as you lower one knee to the side.

✢ Breathe in as you bring the leg back to the center.

✢ Breathe out and lower the other knee to the other side.

✢ Repeat of each side several times.

✢ This exercise stretches everything from the knees to the chest.

I am open and let the good happen.

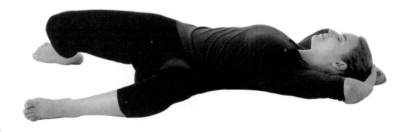

7. Candle 1

❋ Lying on your back, bend your knees and raise your torso onto your shoulders, your hands supporting your lower back.

❋ Straighten your legs and point your toes to the ceiling.

❋ Move both legs in the air as if you are riding a bicycle; bending and straightening.

❋ Remain in this position with one leg elevated for ten to twenty inhalations, saying silently:

*My inner depth is my
highest connection.*

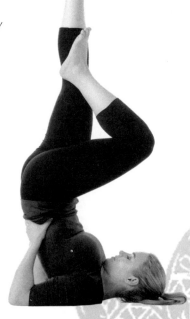

Closing Resting Position

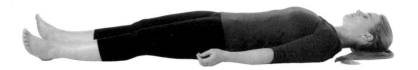

*I wish peace and strength for my
body, spirit, and soul.*

Meditation

The moon represents the element of water. It is the symbol for the emotional realm and the subconscious patterns that have stamped themselves onto your subconsciousness in the past—negative energies, patterns, and moods—and that can make your life difficult. The following meditation frees you from worries, burdens, and weaknesses.

❋ Sit comfortably with your spine straightened or in your preferred meditative pose. Take six deep breaths. With each slow exhale, let all tension go from your face, shoulders, arms, chest, back, pelvis, and legs.

❋ Visualize in your mind's eye: You are sitting on the beach. As you inhale deeply, imagine the water is being pulled toward you, and it gently flows around your pelvis.

❋ As you exhale, the water flows back into a wave, taking with it all of your negativities, pains, burdens, and bad memories. Let everything go with love and attention. Let inner joy and freedom fill you in this new void.

Mantra

Everything in my awareness or in my subconscious that bothers me, I release to the ocean of healing.

Mudra

* Your hands are loose on your lap, the fingers are clasped, except for the pointer fingers, which are pressed together, pointing at the floor, allowing for outward flow.

* The tips of the thumbs lie on two important expulsion points that are then engaged. The stimulation in the pointer fingers activates the large intestine.

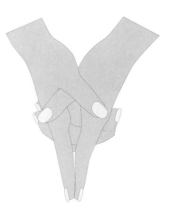

Tuesday

DAY OF MARS

Ancient Nordic people honored their war god, Tyr, with this day (Tyr's Day), as the Romans honored Mars and the Greeks honored Ares. Mars was also the god of gatherings for debate and still today many agricultural exchanges take place on Tuesdays.

Mars embodies the impulsive power of mankind that urges expression and action. This power is neutral; we alone decide how to use it. It gives physical movement to stress in instances of challenge and competition. Mars brings its power to encourage your talents and virtues to flourish. A person must give the offering of talent to Mars or else Mars will look for one to take. The impulsive power of Mars can drive someone to do something they don't want to do or, in some instances, can't do.

The power of Mars helps us to reach our goals physically—as in sports and yoga. In the spiritual realm, Mars helps us concentrate, learn, and build assertive ability and decisiveness. For the soul, Mars evokes excitement, courage, sense of adventure, and belief in yourself.

The negative side to Mars is that it is also responsible for violent temper, anger, impatience, and aggression. The sense of justice belongs to Mars, as well as the fight for justice. Mars strengthens our abilities to decide how much heteronomy we can handle.

Tuesday can be our most productive day at work. On this day we can test our limits and overcome challenges. Tuesday is the ideal day for intensive sports or power yoga. If we are aware of this power and are able to use it, we can reach new levels in our lives.

Exercise routine for motivation

Mars effects our blood, gallbladder, liver, muscles, and male reproductive organs. The following exercise routine strengthens the muscles in the back, shoulders, arms, legs, and stomach. The power of the muscles influences the spiritual and divine sense we carry. They empower desire, stamina, and self esteem. And importantly, using our muscles puts us in a good mood. Later, the exercises of internal motivation are awakened through the circulatory system and gallbladder meridian.

Marching in Place warms the body up and regulates blood pressure. Side Stretches awaken the meridians uniformly.

In the Stretch, Chair, Dog, Paddle Boat, and Bridge, the respective muscles are further strengthened and invigorated.

Tips for throughout the day

- Be aware of your posture while sitting and standing. Maintain a posture that is upright and centered, with shoulders loose.
- Be aware of your movement. It should have a regulated rhythm and powerful tempo.
- Use every chance you have to move your body.

1. Marching in Place

❊ The left knee and right elbow are raised and lowered, followed by the right knee and left elbow. Repeat each cycle with momentum until you are warm. Don't forget to smile!

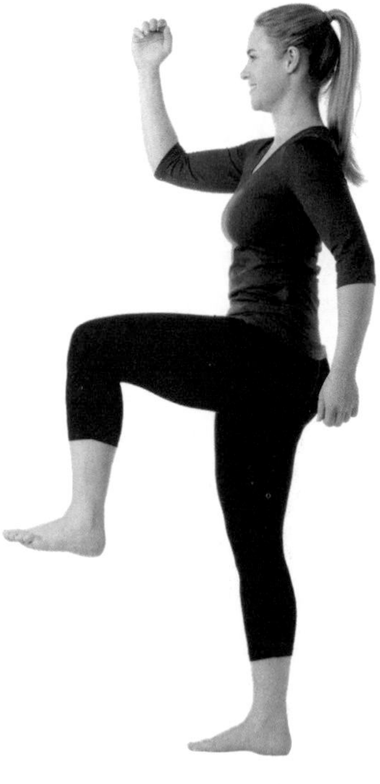

2. Side Stretch

❋ Breathe in and place your right hand on the floor as you raise your left arm high above your head.

❋ Hold your breath as you stretch the entire body toward the right.

❋ Switch sides, and repeat four to six times.

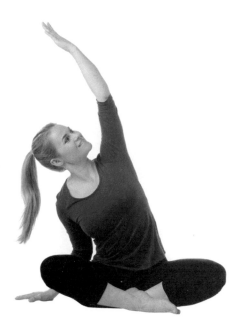

3. Stretch

✳ Stand with your feet shoulder width apart, legs and arms straight, and spread your fingers wide.

✳ Inhale as you stretch one hand to the floor in front of you and raise the opposite hand above you.

✳ Alternate sides, and do six to eight repetitions.

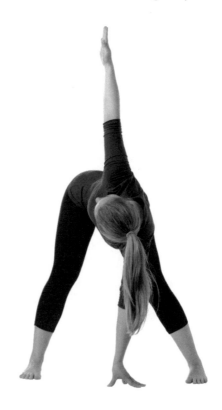

4. Chair

✳ Stand and raise your arms above your head, holding your elbows with your hands.

✳ Inhale and begin to go to a seated position. Hold the position as long as you can.

✳ Repeat four times and end with your body upright and hands on your thighs to start the Dog position on the next page.

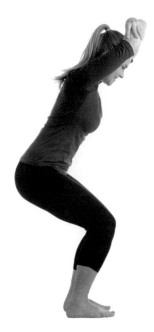

5. Dog

❋ Bend forward from the hips, keeping your arms and legs as straight as possible.

❋ Stretch your torso toward the floor and press your hands firmly on the ground. Your pelvis and rear should be pointed upward. Show the power that resides in you. Growl like a dog—it does you good! Hold as long as you can.

*My power evolves from
each moment to the next.*

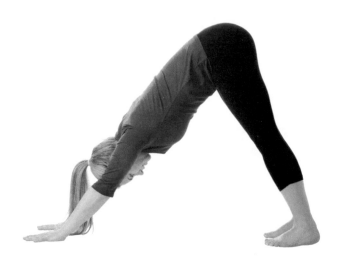

6. Paddle Boat

❊ While sitting on the floor, rest on your forearms and raise your legs up.

❊ Keeping your left leg stretched out, bend your right knee and draw it toward your chest.

❊ Now extend your right leg as you bend the left knee and bring it to your chest.

❊ Alternate and repeat six to ten times.

*I tackle challenges with
joy and vigor.*

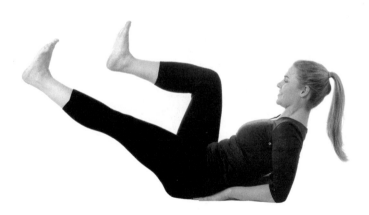

7. Bridge

✵ The Chinese have called this the "energy pump."

✵ Lie on the ground, knees bent, with the soles of your feet pressed flat. Inhale.

✵ Use your buttocks muscles to raise your pelvis upward as you exhale. Your spine thus becomes a burning iron that is forged in warmth.

✵ Hold for as many breaths as is comfortable.

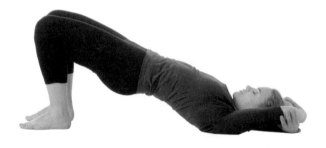

Closing Resting Position

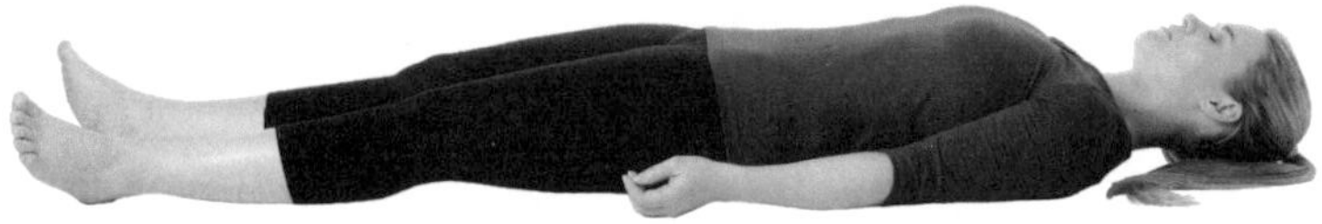

I am aware of my inner strength in my body, spirit, and soul.

Meditation

Mars is associated with fire. In the same way that our body temperature is regulated, so is our temperament. "A fiery temperament" is an expression often used to indicate someone who is hot-headed. This meditation lays the groundwork for a life philosophy: no matter how high and steep our daily challenges, with the right attitude and action, we can reach all summits.

- Sit comfortably on the ground with a straightened spine. Inhale deeply six times.
- Picture in your minds eye: You are at the base of a mountain and are making your way to the top. You are confidently going step by step with ambition in your

stride. You pass by dark rocks, deep ravines, and through beautiful fields. You regularly stop to admire the views.

✳ Integrate the wisdom of this picture and your actions to tackle your daily challenges. You are making it to the top!

Mantra

My fire strengthens every cell in my body,
warms my heart, and heals my spirit.

Mudra

Grab your left middle finger with your right hand and press the right thumb into the left palm. After some time, switch hands.

Two streams of energy run through the middle finger; these are the circulatory and gallbladder meridians. This mudra will awaken them.

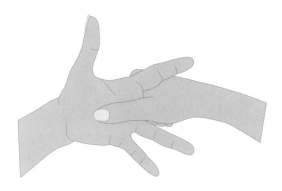

Wednesday

DAY OF MERCURY

Wotan, or Odin, the highest god in the Nordic pantheon, is honored on Wednesday. Wotan is a complicated character: the god of war as well as the god of poetry, the god of trickery and the god of insight. Wotan represents unrest, change of all sorts, turmoil, and exhausting the limits of all things. His refuge is poetry and trade.

Mercury later replaced Wotan as the god of Wednesday. In Mercury we can find the same characteristics as Wotan—language and understanding, structured thinking and decisiveness, as well as a strong business sense. Mercury teaches your inner economist that the smallest expenditure can result in a massive gain!

Mercury recognizes things and gives them names. He symbolizes the the power of thought.

Retrospection can lead to the highest awareness, but applied negatively, it leads to rumination. An endless obsession with pondering problems without searching for an actual solution can leave us with a feeling of hopelessness. But retrospection can also help us to correct past behaviors.

Wednesday is the day in the middle of the week (sometimes called "hump day"), which means Wednesday holds the key to balancing the entire week. Paracelsus observed correctly that "The dose makes the poison"—meaning that proper balance is key. This is also true in our lives; we must decide what we are going to do and what we are going to leave undone.

When we take on too much, want too much, plan too many things at the same time, or have too much to multi-task, our lives can be thrown into disarray. Conversely, if we don't have anything to do, or aren't ambitious for anything and make no plans, then boredom and depression set in. Wednesday is about the constant search for the correct balance, which is a life-long project. More likely than not, once we have found the balance, something new comes along and changes everything. This is the nature of airy Mercury.

On Wednesday we must look at our responsibilities and tasks more clearly. Where in your daily activity can you create more balance with each thing you are doing? Why make a huge deal out of something small, and why overcomplicate things? Are you making mountains out of molehills?

Less is often more.

Exercise routine for mental vigor

Our thinking can be decidedly negatively influenced if the two halves of the brain are not working in tandem or if one side is over-activated or not activated.

Health, satisfaction, and happiness are holistic goals. When our brains are in balance, we can think clearly, with more concentration, sympathy, and creativity. Many yoga exercises are beneficial to brain training. The Wednesday exercises bring spiritual awareness and release serotonin.

Crossover and Standing Cross stimulate the brain; Little Cat is for practicing balance. The Crawl and Chest Mover exercise the spinal column to release and unblock cranial nerves. In Rabbit, the cerebral circulation is optimized. This position in known to yogis as the seat of awareness. In the last position, Quiet Frog, everything is relaxed and tension released.

Tips for throughout the day

❋ Before each challenging daily task, rub your hands together and clap. This increases mental vigor.

❋ Always work in well-ventilated rooms!

❋ Keep hydrated.

❋ Use this power mudra: Clasp your hands together at the back of the head. Point your elbows wide behind you and breathe deeply.

1. Crossover

* Stand with arms to your sides, and breathe in as you put your right leg behind you and stretch your left arm above you.

* Breathe out, bringing your right knee toward your left elbow, touching the elbow tip to the knee.

* Switch sides and repeat six to ten times.

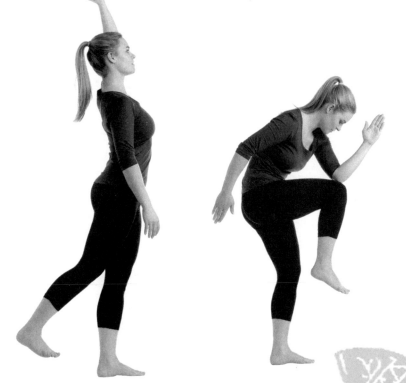

2. Standing Cross

- Raise your arms above your head and stand with your legs and arms crossed—right ankle over left, and right wrist over left. Hold for ten to twelve breaths.
- Change the direction of the cross. Hold for ten to twelve breaths.

The correct dose of everything brings joy and satisfaction.

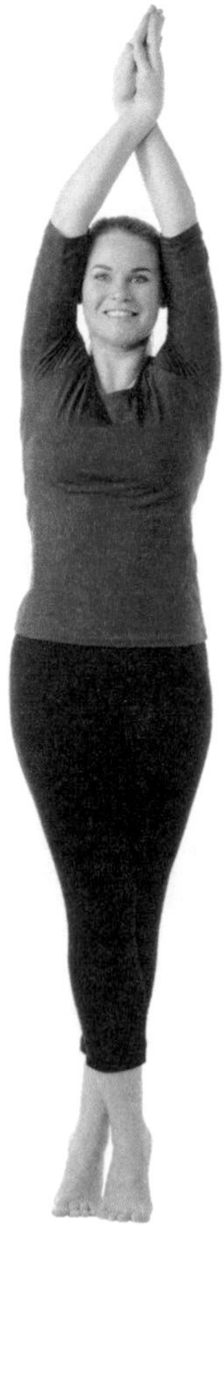

3. Chest Mover

✳ Stand with feet together and palms pressed together in front of your chest.

✳ With matching tempo, move your arms and knees side to side in opposite directions.

✳ Slowly move to and fro twelve times.

✳ Inhale and exhale each time you switch direction.

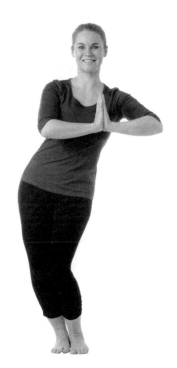

4. The Crawl

✳ On all fours, crawl slowly forward and backward so that one leg moves independently of the other.

✳ While doing so, use an imaginary tail to sway your rear end. (This swaying action may cause your legs to cross each other as a way of balancing yourself as you move forward.)

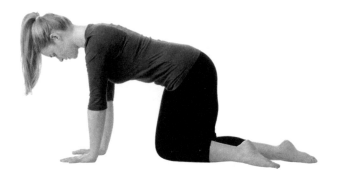

5. The Little Cat

❋ Begin with knees and elbows on the floor.

❋ Inhale as you lift your left arm and left leg.

❋ Exhale as you return your leg and arm to the ground.

❋ Alternate sides, and repeat six times.

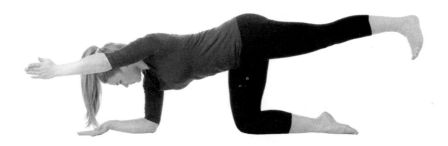

6. The Rabbit

✴ Start by kneeling with your arms hanging loosely by your sides.

✴ Press your chin to your chest.

✴ Lean into the position demonstrated, with your head touching the floor.

✴ Hold for ten to twelve breaths.

Quiet and powerful are my thoughts.

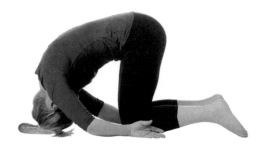

7. The Quiet Frog

✤ Sit on your heels with your knees wide apart so that you can bend forward between your thighs.

✤ With your forearms on the floor, press your forehead on your arms.

✤ With each inhalation, imagine a light entering your body, making it lighter.

✤ Hold for ten to twelve breaths.

*My higher awareness always lets me know
what is wise and what isn't.*

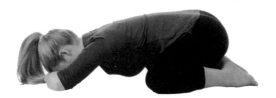

Closing Resting Position

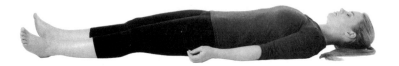

Peace, power, and harmony
fill my entire being.

Meditation

Wednesday is associated with the element of air. The amount of oxygen in the air can affect how we think and change our mental vigor. Everyone can enjoy a nice breeze, but too much forceful movement of the air and it becomes a storm. The same can be said of our thinking. Nervousness, anxiety, impatience, and jumping to conclusions can blow us away from progress. The following meditation (with mudra) brings a peaceful energizing flow to the brain, allowing for connection and activation of both halves of the brain. This allows for deeper concentration and increases creative problem-solving.

* Sit comfortably with a straightened spine or in your usual meditation position.

* Now try the three *bandhas*: Breathe in and tighten the anal muscle, tighten your diaphragm all the way to the chin and in the throat.

* Stay in this pose for a few seconds and release the tension as you exhale.

* Repeat up to ten times.

Mantra

In all places and at all times I am aware—what I think in my mind becomes my reality.

Mudra

Spread your fingers apart, touching the fingertips of each hand.

This finger position synchronizes the two halves of the brain and deepens the breath.

*Good friends and small parties
are the spice of life.*

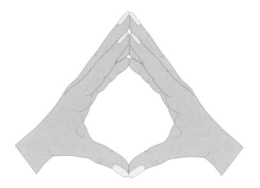

Thursday

DAY OF JUPITER

Thursday is named in honor of the Nordic god Thor. He was very popular, a muscle man, blusterer, a beer drinker with an insatiable appetite. Thor rarely had to fight since his aggressive reputation preceded him. In the astrological sense, Jupiter represents the exact same qualities, which in turn leaves Thursday as the manifestation of Jupiter.

Jupiter's power allows us to feel the larger sense of life, the wisdom that life isn't arbitrary but is meaningful, that life is better understood as being eternal and transcendental. When we are aware that life brings challenges, joy, suffering, and deeper meaning, then our inner strength can unfurl and reach out to protect us from the bad and take in the good. If we are met with sorrow or tragedy, the experience can be more easily taken in with the understanding that a larger plan is involved. Jupiter represents the ubiquitous motto: "This too shall pass."

We all carry the desire to have a joyful life; to strive for joy is a human necessity that creates lasting wellness and a well-rounded life. Jupiter represents these desires in us. Jupiter is playful and likes raucous festivities and everything that raises our sense of the joy of living.

Jupiter is adored far and wide as being tolerant and courageous, as well as generous, loving, and giving. Nothing is demure in Jupiter's nature! Jupiter is gallant down to each and every detail.

Thursday, Thor's day, is the ideal day to connect with your inner sense of Jupiter. Jupiter loves being social, so why not make this a time to build new friendships or take care of existing ones? This could mean something as simple as a phone call or email or a dinner out with a friend and a good glass of wine.

Thursday used to be known as "little Sunday," a time when people would eat better foods and drink more than usual to get the most out of life. Thursday is the ideal day to celebrate and enjoy.

Exercises for digestion

Tension and issues with the digestive system are very common in our modern age. Problems can include gastric illnesses, bloating, cramps, and a feeling of being unwell. These can be ameliorated by stretching the belly area through the Belly and Stomach Stretch, in which the inner and outer stomach is stretched and compacted. This increases blood flow to allow more nourishment to the organs, helping them to become strong and regular.

The position Hop warms up and relaxes the diaphragm. Stomach Inversion is a well-known yoga exercise that releases tension in the body's core allowing for increased circulation throughout entire body.

The effects of Leaf bring the circulation all the way into the fists and have the same tension relieving benefits as Stomach Inversion. In Side Stretches the liver, spleen, and intestines get a good workout. In this version of the Crocodile, the pose massages the stomach area, and the Candle pose again increases the blood flow.

Tips for throughout the day

- Healthy food doesn't have to be expensive or complicated. A vegetable dish is easy to make. Meat and fish intake should be reduced and fresh fruit should be eaten.

- Plan healthy menus ahead of time that you like to make and are worth it! Your body will certainly know what you are doing and thank you. Don't forget to try something new now and again.

1. Hop

✳ Hop in place from foot to foot with your arms raised
   loosely above your head. Keep this up for as long as
   feels comfortable, but not so long as to make you feel
   winded. This exercise energizes and warms up the body,
   increasing the blood flow.

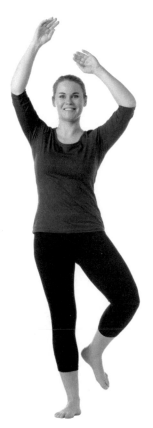

2. Stomach Inversion

❋ On your hands and knees, breathe in and raise your head.

❋ Exhale and lower your head, drawing your chin inward toward your chest. Inhale.

❋ Breathe out while arching your back upward as far as you comfortably can. This allows for deeper breathing on your next inhale.

❋ Raise your head again while you deeply inhale.

❋ Repeat six times.

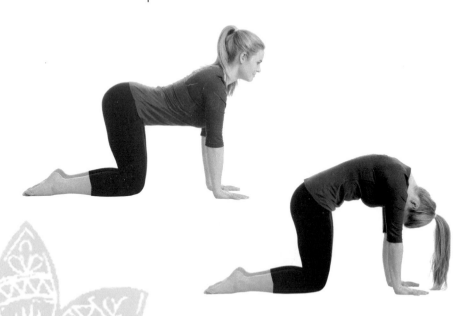

3. Belly and Stomach Stretch

✽ Sit on your knees with your hands, palm side down, on
the floor behind you.

✽ Raise your torso and hold your neck and head straight
while looking directly forward.

✽ Hold the pose for ten to twelve breaths.

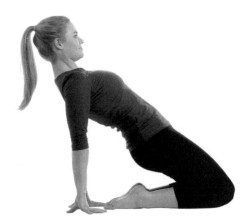

4. Leaf

❋ Kneel and sit on the backs of your legs, as shown in the position below.

❋ Ball your fists and press them on your stomach, just above your navel.

❋ Lean forward and rest your head on the ground.

❋ Hold for ten to twelve breaths.

I am completely thankful
for my enriched life.

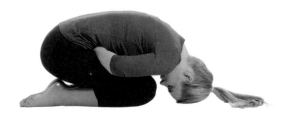

5. Side Stretches and Knee Stand

✳ Position yourself as shown, with your body supported by your left knee on the floor and your right leg bent with your foot on the floor.

✳ Stretch your left arm over your head, turning your head to the left. Your right arm can rest on your right thigh. You should feel a stretch through your left torso.

✳ Hold this pose for fifteen breaths.

✳ Change position to the opposite leg and repeat the exercise.

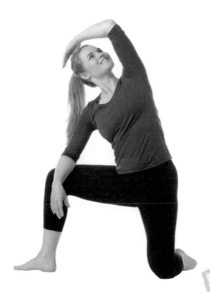

6. Crocodile 2

✳ Begin by lying on your back, with your knees bent and raised toward your chest. Rest your arms on the floor, hands above your head and elbows bent.

✳ Breathe out, lowering your knees together to one side while turning your head in the opposite direction toward your elbow.

✳ Breathe in, bringing your knees back to the middle, returning your head to center.

✳ Change sides: breathe out and lower your legs to the opposite side, turning your head to face the opposite elbow.

✳ Alternate sides, repeating eight times.

I release myself to the waves of change with ease.

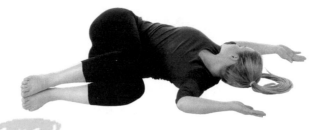

7. Candle 2

✳ Lying on your back, bend your knees and raise yourself onto your shoulders, your hands supporting your lower back.

✳ Straighten your legs and point your toes to the ceiling.

✳ Move your legs and feet together in a small movement, creating a figure 8, until you feel your stomach being massaged.

I bring peace and power to my center.

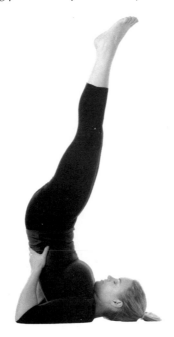

Closing Resting Position

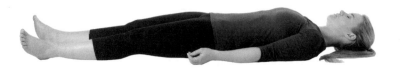

*I am open to the good
and am open for it to fill my life.*

Meditation

Jupiter is associated with space, unending time, and the higher planes of existence. Jupiter directly affects our futures. We influence our futures unconsciously with our imaginations, our thoughts, and our feelings.

The following meditation will allow you to bring your thoughts into a positive energy flow. Imagine all of your wishes with complete fervor, but don't forget to also be physically relaxed as you do.

* Sit with a straightened back or in your preferred meditation position. Take six deep breaths.

* Imagine you are looking at a movie screen onto which you are projecting a film. In this film, you are the lead actor and in control of the future. You look happy, healthy, and full of satisfaction. You are doing what you want to do surrounded by supportive and well-meaning people. Feel that you are 100 percent of yourself and have the lead. Look around you at the place where you are and the people you are with. Your positivity brings joy to them all and fills the space entirely.

* Think about this scene before you got to bed and when you wake up. Have fun!

Mantra

*I open myself to the gifts of life—
my heart is full of joy and goodness.*

Mudra

Your pinky finger and index finger are pointed straight out. Your middle and ring fingers together are pressed inward on your thumbs. This mudra is good for digestion and increases the flow of energy to your body's core.

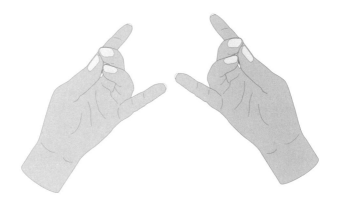

Friday

DAY OF VENUS

riday is named for the Germanic goddess Frigga, more formally known as consort of Odin. She is the goddess of love, fertility, and of women. She is the representation of beauty, wisdom, and the force of love. These virtues also belong to the Roman goddess Venus.

Beauty excites us, drives us, and brings us luck. It awakens a deep passion in us that reflects our divine perfection. Venus represents harmony and opens us to the realms of color and sound. The polar opposite is also within us—discord and tension. Venus symbolizes the need for harmony and a reduction of tension and opposes negative influences to our equilibrium.

Venus requires from us only that we enjoy our personal beauty and indulge in enjoying everything in life that is harmonious and pleasing. Indulging in the beauty that is life will lead to peace and awaken new powers within us.

Venus loves enchantment, both actively (in which you enchant and turn the heads of everyone in the room), as well as passively (in which you yourself are enchanted).

We should be careful when indulging in beauty that we don't fall into the trap of narcissism. Narcissistic infatuation means being indulged by others without reciprocation. We must be sure not to become spellbound by this principle, which Venus can awaken.

Sympathy, empathy, and antipathy are always in the realm of indulgence. We must be mindful that what we are drawn toward is in our best interests. In other words, welcome the indulgence of Venus, but let your awakening inner awareness help you decide what is best to let into your life.

On Friday, you will do yourself a world of good to indulge in something that is beautiful after a long and productive week. Friday is a day for a nice scented bath, a bouquet of flowers, a visit to an art museum, and even some nice chocolates! And it is certainly a day for a romantic candlelit dinner or a fun night out with friends.

Exercise routine for relaxation

Venus influences our balance, the female reproductive organs, the kidneys, the vascular system, and respiratory glands. Venus stands for harmony, comfort, beauty, and love. The yoga exercises on this day will aide the kidneys, adrenal glands, and hormone production; working on these systems promotes feelings of comfort, courage, and love.

The Loose Arm Swing is meant for general relaxation and warming up. Pendulum strengthens balance, and relaxes the shoulders. Pyramid invigorates the neck and stabilizes the legs. Side Balance promotes relaxation. With these positions, we are utilizing the muscles and ligaments that we seldom use in our daily lives.

In the positions Grasshopper and Cobra, we bring energy in our entire back to later be released in Turtle. These final three positions will create a flushing flow of energy to the kidneys.

Tips for throughout the day

✻ Let yourself daydream and enjoy nice thoughts anytime and anywhere; research suggests that this is good for our health!

✻ Think of where and how can you show your love, respect, and support throughout the day. Don't put it off any longer—Friday is the ideal day for such indulgences.

1. Loose Arm Swing

❋ Swing both arms together to the right and to the left in a smooth movement; as you swing them, trace a figure eight on its side.

❋ Inhale to the right; exhale to the left.

❋ End by raising your arms up to the right and to the left several times.

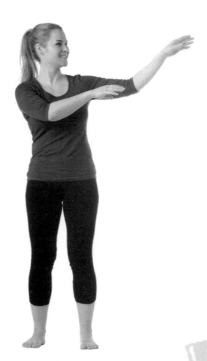

2. Pendulum

∗ Stand on your left leg with your left hand on your front pelvic bone

∗ With your right arm and right leg, make small circles in the air (as many as feel comfortable—you'll be able to do more circles as your balance improves and your core strengthens).

∗ Repeat several times on both sides.

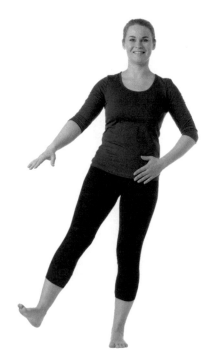

3. Pyramid

✳ Stand with your feet pointing straight ahead at a width just past your shoulders.

✳ Bending from your hips and keeping your legs straight, reach your arms between and behind your legs. Your palms should face down.

✳ Stay in this position for ten to twenty breaths and focus your mind on something beautiful.

I want to discover the beauty in everything.

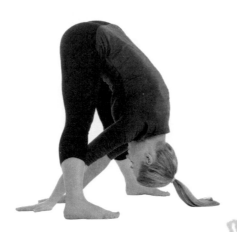

4. Side Balance

❊ Lie on your left side as shown with your left arm and left leg fully extended.

❊ Inhale and raise your right arm and right leg in the air, perpendicular to your body.

❊ Exhale and lower the arm and leg.

❊ Repeat ten times, then switch sides and repeat another ten times.

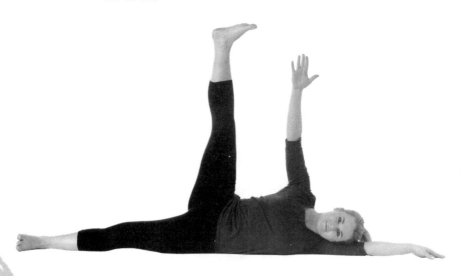

5. Grasshopper

✳ Lie on your stomach with your pelvic bones resting on both hands.

✳ Inhale and raise your right leg.

✳ Exhale and lower your leg.

✳ Switch legs and repeat.

✳ Alternate raising and lowering each leg six times.

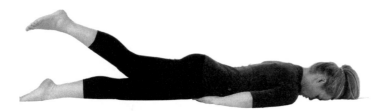

6. Cobra

❋ A similar position as the Grasshopper, but your hands are behind you, cupping your buttocks.

❋ Inhale as you raise your upper torso, and exhale as you lower it.

❋ Repeat four times.

❋ Finish by staying in the raised position as long as you can.

The cobra brings me power,
courage and self trust.

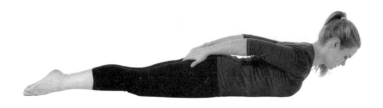

7. Turtle

❋ Similar to the Pyramid, but with a sitting posture instead
of a standing posture.

❋ Sit on your heels and lower your head to the ground as
you stretch your arms back between your legs toward
your feet.

❋ Keep your hands, palms out, between your feet and hold
the position for ten to twenty breaths.

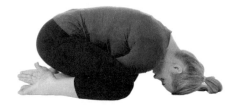

Closing Resting Position

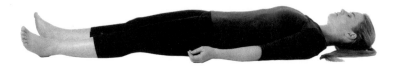

I am open to all beauty and I open myself to receive it everywhere in my life.

Meditation

When we direct all our senses toward beauty, we strengthen ourselves on every level. Beauty is nourishment for the soul. It creates harmony and balance within us, and thus harmony and balance in all our bodily functions. Engage your senses more often to consciously hear, see, smell, taste, and feel beauty in all its forms. Becoming more attuned to beauty will support and stimulate your sensuousness—your life—to be richer and bolder.

The following exercise regenerates and calls upon our inner power in order to create a feeling of "time out" during your day.

* Sit in a comfortable position with a straightened spine or in your preferred meditation position. Take six deep breaths.

* In your mind's eye, imagine you are looking at a wonderful place (real or imagined) that speaks to your sense of beauty, peace, and harmony—a place where you would like to spend a minute, a day, a week.

* Breathe in the air in this place and enjoy the aroma; look at the shapes and colors of this place; try to *hear* what this place sounds like—birds singing, wind, water, music—the sound of earthly or heavenly angels. You are completely relaxed; all is good.

Mantra

Peace, harmony, and beauty rule my life.

Mudra

Cup both hands by pressing the ring fingers and thumbs together. Keep this position with your hands on your lap.

This finger position activates the flow of energy in the kidneys and liver. It acts against melancholy and feelings of inner emptiness and loneliness. You awaken the creativity of the sun. The ring finger corresponds to Apollo the Sun God, and the grooves on the ring finger speak to Venus, a truly compatible pair.

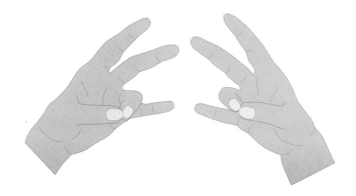

Saturday

DAY OF SATURN

Saturday is Saturn's day. In astrology, Saturn can be a dark companion whose strength and earnestness can besiege us. But Saturn can also protect us from many things that tempt us, things that may harm us. Saturn is a protector as well as a force for change.

The virtues of Saturn are stamina, stability, durability, discernment, perfectionism, and concentration. Saturn provides the endurance—the power—to see something through to empower our lives. Its confers the quality of reservation that allows us to keep things to ourselves. Because Saturn represents the ability to discern and analyze, its power allows us to purge our lives of what we do not need. This does not mean that we have to wall ourselves off from the world—that would be lonely—but rather it endows us with the ability to figure out what is good and bad for us.

Saturn gives us the ability to debunk old patterns and ways of thinking; to cast off materialism and the constant need to want more. Saturn gives power to our concentration so that we may spend our mental energy on that which is most important.

Saturn also belongs to the realm of fate and the feeling that we don't have control over our path in life. This is a feeling that can overpower us and create negative emotions. It can ruin our chances of finding solutions to our problems—"I think there is a higher power making a plan, and my life path is already in place."

However, our lives are not hard because of the circumstances we face; life can be easy or hard based on how we approach our situation. We all face changes in our lives that we feel are out of our control. Saturn's energy can show us a way through by teaching us to look inside, be introspective, and determine how to let go and what we should cast off and leave behind.

Retrospection can be helpful and good for us, but only when it is used to learn from our past mistakes. Very often retrospection turns into rumination—a futile rethinking of what could have been. One of Saturn's most important functions is to teach us to discern between healthy retrospection and anxiety-producing rumination.

Saturn represents what is being hidden and not shown to the world, but Saturn also provides the introspection required to bring things into the light so that we may grow and develop. Saturn teaches us that inaction is often as necessary as action.

Saturn promotes cleanliness and refinement. Saturday is often the day we set aside for chores and housework, or home improvement projects. On Saturday you can clean externally *and* internally; look back on the week and see what was holding you back, what was unnecessary, and what helped propel you forward. Saturday is the day to review the week, and then expel it from your mind.

Exercises for flexibility

Saturn affects our bones and our joints. By moving a single joint with concentration, slowly tightening and relaxing it, you can change your metabolism. Working the cartilage in the joints can produce a huge change in us by feeding the joints and cleaning them! Regular movement keeps our ligaments elastic and durable.

We begin the following exercise series with Plucking Stars to warm up. After that, each subsequent pose works selected joints, wherein each are systematically and consciously moved eight times. During each pose, you should feel the joint that you're moving and visualize sending it reinvigorating light to optimize the effects.

Tips for throughout the day

✻   It doesn't matter if you are standing, sitting, or lying down.

✻   Use any down time or waiting time to move one or two of your joints with concentration.

1. Plucking Stars

❋ Reach one hand at a time as high as you can toward the sky. Stretch so that you can pluck a star out of the heavens. (This star represents something you have wished for.)

 ❋ Bring this star, with intention, to your heart and feel its energy.

 ❋ Alternating sides, repeat ten times.

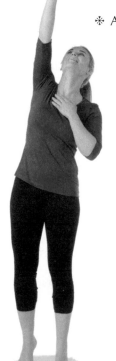

2. Bird in the Nest

- Stand as shown on one leg, knee slightly bent.
- Raise your other leg behind you, lowering your head and torso. Try to keep your body and leg in the same plane.
- Palms down, extend your arms behind your shoulders.
- Move your wrists and the raised ankle joint in a small circular motion. Make at least eight rotations of the ankle joint.
- Repeat on other side, with another eight ankle rotations.

Anything that is a burden to me, I cast off
and enjoy the ease I feel.

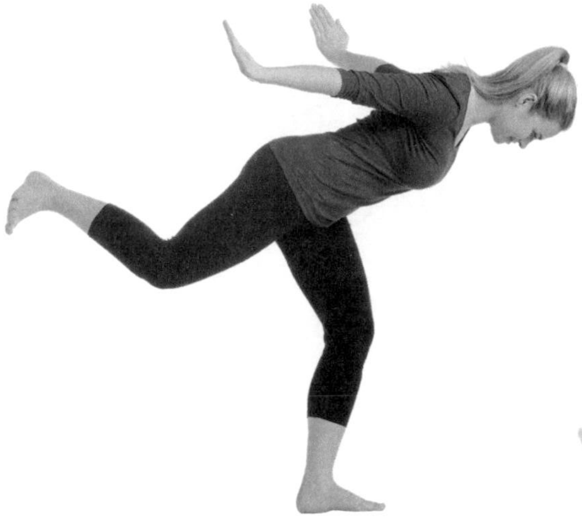

3. Arm Bends and Stretches

❋ Sit with your buttocks on your legs.

❋ Inhale and stretch out your arms, fingers interlaced, palms facing away.

❋ Exhale and bend your arms inward toward your chest. Keep your elbows at shoulder height.

❋ Repeat eight times

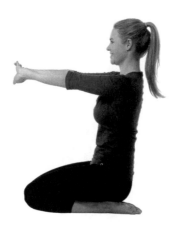

4. Arm Circles (Shoulder Joint)

❋ Lie on your left side with your left leg and left arm extended.

❋ Bring your right knee toward your chest. With the right arm completely loose, make a slow circular motion.

❋ Switch to the other side and repeat.

❋ Do this exercise eight times on each side.

I open my heart to the treasures of the future.

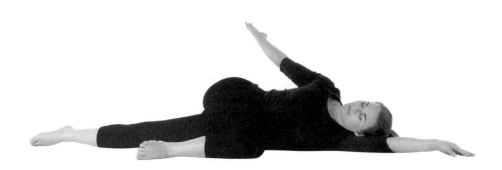

5. Leg Circles (Hip Joint)

* Lie on your back with your legs on the floor.

* Bring one leg, knee bent, toward your chest, and with
  an exhale, raise the opposite leg, stretching it toward the
  ceiling.

* Inhale, and bring the raised leg slowly down and toward
  your chest, then raise it upward again as you exhale.

* Do eight repetitions, and switch to the other leg and
  repeat.

Everything passes by and I keep going.

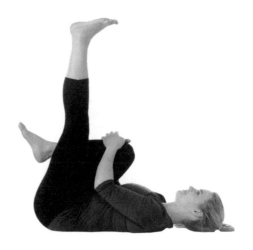

6. Candle 3 (Knees)

✳ Assume the Candle Pose (page 39), raised up on your shoulders with your hands supporting your lower back.

✳ With your feet about shoulder width apart, lower both legs toward your head (exhale) and then straighten them (inhale) toward the ceiling.

✳ Repeat eight times

My self assurance empowers me.

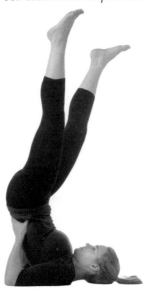

7. Little Bear

✽ Lying on your back with all limbs straightened and
pointing upward, flex your wrists and ankles in circles
until you begin to feel tired.

I love myself just as I am.

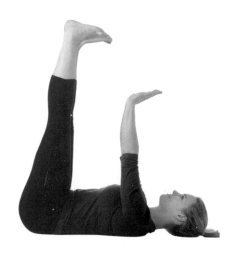

Closing Resting Position

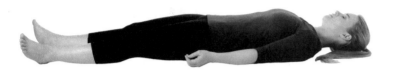

Freedom, joy, and liberty fill my body, spirit, and soul.

Meditation

Saturn is usually thought of in connection with the morning and dawn. Just as the night is at its darkest and can seem hopeless, full of loneliness and confusion, Saturn comes in as a harbinger to the Sun, which brings light and hope to the day.

Sunrise is like a gate. This is an image often seen in fairy tales: the hero or heroine standing at the gate as the sun rises, having solved the riddle or overcome the challenge and now facing the opening day with a pure heart. So is it in our lives: each day opens to a new scene, a new possibility, and with it comes the new challenges that will change and shape us.

On Saturday, take the time to ask for wisdom to be present and to be active throughout your day, and the coming week.

✳ Sit comfortably with a straightened spine or in your preferred meditation position.

✳ Take six deep breaths.

✳ Imagine that you are on a trip or a long journey or even a religious pilgrimage. You pack your backpack, but only what you truly need.

✳ You come to a gate—a symbol for a crossing and a passage toward a new world and a new time. Here you beseech your wisdom: What must I do? What must I let go of to allow sense and joy into my future at this place and in my new life there?

✳ Stay in the pose and after a short time the answer will come to you.

Mantra

I am as I am, I love myself as I am and I always make the best of what I am. I accept life as it is, I respect life as it is, and I always make the best of it.

Mudra

Interlock your thumbs and index fingers of both hands with other fingers laced together. Now, keep your hands at the top of your abdomen.

This mudra calms you on many levels and brings a sense of completeness—even with your weaknesses and strengths. When we bring ourselves to this acceptance, we increase our self-trust and wisdom.

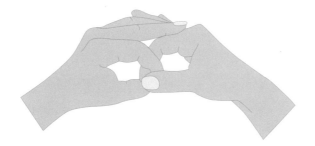

SEVEN
MAGICAL WEEKS

Every day brings a new beginning, full of possibilities. With every day we have another opportunity to create a plan that allows for our optimal happiness. We can't change our lives in monumental ways at once, but we can make the best of every single moment, day by day.

This daily step-by-step approach also applies to individual weeks. When we have become accustomed to planning and directing our days in a metaphysical manner, we can also do the same for the weeks of the year. As you have seen, each day of the week is devoted to a different body system, using the energies represented by the daily planetary correspondences. Once you have set up a routine and become comfortable with your daily practice, start thinking in terms of weeks.

In my own daily practice, I have become aware that small efforts—even as small as seven minutes—can bring enormous change both in character and in circumstances. Through yoga practice, our gifts and talents are nurtured to benefit and improve our lives. Practicing yoga, meditation, mantras, and mudras through the days and over weeks, I became more and more aware of my own flaws and talents. For instance, I became aware of my tendency to always be running late, thus making both myself and those around me stressed. As a result of this insight, I decided to dedicate a weekly yoga cycle in which I made a conscious effort to not be rushed and during which I had to honestly pay attention to the time. Through this, I have learned to take on no more and no less than I can handle on a daily basis.

We can simply let the weeks fly by with no plan and no goal, or we can plan out weeks in advance to concentrate on those qualities that need to be honed to better our lives.

With this in mind, I have created seven weekly themes to make a cycle that you can follow and repeat throughout the year. Incorporating this pattern into your yogic practice is easy and requires little thought. It is really as simple as focusing your intention on the following themes. For example, the mantra for Sunday practice is *"I open myself to the divine joy, may I be filled with it through my heart as I go into the world."* During week one, you will add the underlying concept of organization to your intention. And so on for each of the days in week one.

The physical poses that we do in yoga are one thing; the deeper meaning of these poses is what creates the great spiritual development that unfolds. These deeper meanings are what I have presented in the weekly themes.

Week 1: Organization

Week 2: Focus

Week 3: Creativity

Week 4: Analysis

Week 5: Generosity

Week 6: Celebration

Week 7: Spirituality

The number one goal of practice is the development of personal consciousness and its connection with universal consciousness.

Week 1

ORGANIZATION

riedrich Nietzsche said, "One must still have chaos in oneself to be able to give birth to a dancing star." This quote is a consolation for those who prefer order in their lives but somehow can't seem it pull it all together. However, we have learned from various studies that people who were put in painfully organized rooms were less creative than when they were put it rooms that were cluttered. Researchers found that creative inspiration was five times more likely to occur in places with a little chaos.

We've all had the experience that our best ideas happen when we don't have time for them. And when we do eventually have the time or place to come up with good ideas, the impulse, insight, or feeling is no longer there.

Being organized means taking into account both order and chaos. You cannot really control either. It is important to have a writing pad close by (or use the notepad on your cell phone) so that you can jot down any ideas that might suddenly come to you—or else you will lose them forever.

Focusing on the concept of organization will allow you to create space for, and be prepared for, the new and unknown to come into your life. Spiritual "rearrangement" can take place once we make space for it by casting off the old, the unused, and the unnecessary. Allow a little bit of unplanned chaos to enter your life! Inner reorganization will eventually lead to enrichment of your creative self.

A little bit of planning for this is like magic. You clean your closet and kitchen cabinets, but you should also reorganize your planner, your contact list, and all old information and files on your computer.

There is another reason why disposing of old matters is so important. Most things that we hoard in our homes are connected with the past and keep us there. Patanjali speaks of this in the Yoga Sutras when he says that these old connections bring with them a painful aura. With such negative memories we must think, where are the good memories? Recognize that what made bad memories in the past will make bad experiences now.

What are you still holding on to that is really no good for you? Know what those things are so you can avoid making the same errors. Reorganize! And then don't look back; move forward with nothing holding you back.

Only when you travel with a light pack will you easily arrive at your destination and enjoy the lightness of life.

This week you cast off what holds you back, you reorganize. Keep the lesson in mind that a little chaos is good for us!

Week 2

FOCUS

This week is all about focusing your thoughts. Focusing is not the same thing as concentrating; it means directing our thoughts with intention. Our thoughts create our reality and thus have everything to do with our future and with creating happiness and joy.

Carefully examine your thoughts and link them to the flow of what is dear to you. Our thinking can become habitual—this means we let our thought patterns become stuck on the same path and our brains cannot develop in new directions. For example, when we are sick and finally get well, our thoughts might still circle around the fear of becoming ill again. Similarly, some people are not able to let go of their ex; some people are not able to leave their work at the office. We can spoil our daily lives thinking like this—when our thoughts are unfocused we do not enjoy the present, and we may end up poorly constructing our future.

Unfocused thoughts can also make us physically ill; they weaken our immune system and create stress for our internal organs. We have to learn to bridle our negative thoughts and refocus them onto the positive, because our thoughts do indeed create our reality. The thing you fear, the thing that causes stress, heartache, or anxiety, is not *outside* you. Reality and your thoughts are not separate—your thoughts *are* your reality. Learn to focus them.

When we don't pay attention, negative thought patterns can take over. So how can we free ourselves from this?

Accept the fact that you are constantly thinking and that you will be consumed with whatever you are thinking about. During this week of focus, use the following tip to make yourself more aware of your thoughts. Put this note in your bathroom, on your kitchen counter, on your computer: "What are you thinking about?" Stop for a moment when you see these notes, focus on your current thought, and, if necessary, refocus your thought to something positive. You will then suddenly notice that you are thinking in a whole new way.

Week 3

CREATIVITY

*H*ow often have you had the inspiration to start something new but were stymied by the fact that you had to rush off to do something else? We never seem to have time for ourselves. A friend of mine says, "Everyone has their working space, which can be compared to a garden. If you leave your garden untended, it will become overgrown with weeds and nothing new can grow." A garden (you) has to be tended to and weeds removed regularly or creativity will not grow.

Everyone has a talent and fondness for certain things, and this has its place in the higher order of your spiritual self—even if you don't "see" that self or understand it. When our spiritual self is not balanced and in harmony—when we aren't satisfied or happy—we cannot access our talents. We have the feeling that something is missing, or that we missed the chance for something.

My personal experience has taught me that our talents are not simply ours for personal use but rather meant to be used for the greater good. Our personal creativity adds to the creativity of the world around us, increasing joy for all.

Organize this week so that you have a little time for yourself each day. Move any appointments or responsibilities that aren't of a life-or-death nature. Now look at your newly created time slot with joy! Leave this time for doing what you really like to do, like a hobby or something that truly interests you.

Keep in mind that creativity doesn't come from thin air. Creativity isn't about your perfecting something but rather about your doing something that makes you happy, which in turn adds to the greater universal happiness and joy.

Week 4

ANALYSIS

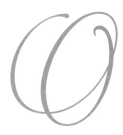ur society can be sorted into two categories: people who have too much to do, and people who don't have enough to do. In which category would you put yourself?

A friend may tell you that they are overwhelmed and have way too much going on, and you think to yourself, "How do they always get into this position? Why can't they simply take on less?" Well from your point of view on the outside, you have the answer and know exactly what to do. But can you do the same for yourself?

Only one thing can help: the analytical week in which all responsibilities are looked at carefully.

During your practice this week, ask yourself the following questions:

Is this responsibility really necessary, or have I simply taken it on out of habit and without thinking about it carefully?

Can I see a way to make this chore easier? Is there a way to delegate what needs to be done? Or am I a control freak who has to do everything myself?

Am I being manipulated? (Tyrants and manipulators come at us from every angle and lay traps.) Can I avoid traps, or do I fall right in?

Am I possibly taking on so many things that I am constantly beginning lots of them but not finishing them? Rather than focusing on what's necessary or important to me, am I texting and chatting on the phone, reading tabloids, or simply zoning out in front of the computer or television?

Remember during this week of analysis that it is important to differentiate between important and unimportant, wise and unwise. And you'll need to dig up your sense of humor and look at yourself and your life with a bit of levity.

Week 5

GENEROSITY

enerosity begins with you. When I see someone who appears to be very generous—giving
gifts and picking up tabs—but who keeps
those around them on a short leash, then I
must question their intentions. You certainly
know the types of people I mean!

During your week of generosity, begin by asking yourself:
How generous am I to *myself*? Where am I not generous? Where
are the limitations of my generosity—and why? What do I like
the most about myself? Where am I wasteful?

This week you give generosity a close look, and wastefulness is the other side of the generosity coin. Where you are
wasteful might be very telling and can make you aware of a
lack of generosity you didn't see before. Here is an example
of how wastefulness hinders your generosity: Small things can
build up in your mind and you can't let go of any of them. This
leads to being bewildered and being overly critical of yourself.
Unless you have a problem with a clear solution, this is wasteful

thinking. Your thoughts are stuck on you—what do you have left to give to others?

I want to make it clear that most self-centered people have an enormous number of small things swirling in their minds and being generous doesn't seem to fit in anywhere. And there are also those people who are being generous only because they want something in return. All of this is very normal in humanity. Therefore we should learn to look at what we consider generous and frugal in ourselves.

Use this week to understand what it means to be generous to yourself and to others. What would be best is to give yourself a gift, something that will make you happy. Now give someone else a gift—it will make you even happier.

Week 6

CELEBRATION

We can always find a reason to celebrate, find hundreds of reasons to reward, and thousands of reasons to be thankful. In most countries, people live a very modest life but there is a lot of celebration. Celebration as I talk about it here doesn't mean the elaborate wedding or party; celebration is simply an outpouring of joy, of thanks, of recognition for life's beauties.

Celebrating always does us good as long as stress isn't part of the celebration. When we celebrate, our thoughts are directed to something joyful and fun. You can celebrate alone, with another person, or with all your friends and acquaintances. It can be as simple or as elaborate as you want—but no stress allowed!

During this week of celebration, think about the following: what do you need to do to create a celebratory feeling? This is a positive emotion that makes us feel happy. Do you celebrate by wearing pretty clothes? With beautiful decorations? With flowers, nice food, wine? What for you creates the feeling of celebration?

When we're down in the dumps, a little celebration can pick up our spirits. Don't you always feel better after a shower, when you have put on nice clothes, and made yourself up? Sometimes just setting a beautiful dinner table can be mood lifting and make a simple daily meal feel like a celebration.

Use this week to create the feeling of thankfulness and being happy for everything. Make as many of your daily routines as you can into mini-celebrations. Feeding your cats? Make a little party of the occasion, sing them songs, dance a little jig. You feel better already, don't you?

We should make small little celebrations as often as we can in our lives. It doesn't matter where or with however many people. You should reward yourself and thank your body for all that it does for you to keep you healthy and happy.

Week 7

SPIRITUALITY

You don't have to spend this week in a monastery or ashram, nor do you have to sit for hours on end in meditation. Outwardly, there is nothing you need to do.

For many years I have been reading the biographies of Christian mystics and Indian ascetics who had insight into enlightenment. I was interested in finding out what made their lives spiritual. I saw many similarities between the Eastern and Western ideals of spirituality and vowed to incorporate them in my daily life. Here is what I found:

First: There is divinity in everything and therefore everything needs to revered and respected. These mystics and seers saw no difference between rich and poor, educated and uneducated.

Second: It doesn't matter what you are physically doing in life; in your heart of hearts you can always connect with the universal consciousness.

Third: Live in the here and now, and trust that the future will take care of itself. There should be a childlike sense of joy as you let go of the fear of the unknown.

Fourth: Take your responsibilities seriously. Carefully fulfill your duties. Don't think of anything as beneath you. Everything you do is for the veneration of the Divine and in service to humanity. Give without expectation of thanks or recognition.

When I read about spiritually enlightened people, it was clear that personal rituals were crucial to their development. Maybe you can set aside a small corner in your house or apartment for this purpose—a place to meditate or practice yoga. Put up pictures or statues that remind you of divinity. In this week of spirituality, take time to do something meaningful to bring you closer to the Divine.

Conclusion

OUR LIFE PHASES

Minutes, days, weeks, months, years. Step by step, moment by moment, we pass through the many phases of life. We have a choice in how to make the best use of our time as we progress through our lives, and I hope this book has provided you a path for taking seven minutes every day and turning those minutes into a lifetime philosophy of health, wellness, and joy.

As a lifelong student of yoga, I have made the observation that life phases are looked at differently in the West and in the East. In the West, we look at our life phases physically—that is, according to time and aging—and in the East, life phases are seen more in terms of philosophy—that is, according to spiritual growth.

In the Western view, the first life phase is the personal development of the child, then the academic development of the young adult, then the family and career development of adulthood, and finally the well-deserved retirement phase, which can last as long as thirty years. In the West, a philosophical view of the life phase often does not occur until retirement, when one is looking back on life.

The Eastern view of life phases is in line with yogic philosophy—as one develops, there can be many paths to choose to follow until one finally comes to rest. Life phases are not so much marked by physical development as they are by spiritual development.

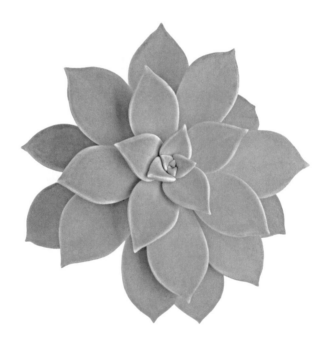

No one life phase should be easier or harder than another. In the West, we tend to think of what we're going to do for ourselves "when we retire"; in other words, when we have time for ourselves. It shouldn't matter what age we are; ask yourself the question *now*: "What patterns am I ready to let go of." Think of three and immediately work to let them go and move forward.

Think of your current strengths. Ask yourself: "What can I do with these at this time, and how can I move forward with them?" Identify three strengths and make sure you put them into action this week, this month.

Make a motto for the next seven years of your life, a motto that encapsulates your dreams, your desires, your divinity, your joy. Consecrate this with a special ritual as a reminder of what you are doing and where you want to go.

DAILY CORRESPONDENCES

Day	Planet	Body System	Yoga Exercises
Sunday	Sun	Heart and circulatory system	Windmill, Arm Rotator, and Chest Twist, Blade, Oak, St. Andrew's Cross, Chest Expander
Monday	Moon	Lymph and water balance systems	Bamboo, Butterfly, Side Arch, Broth Mixer, Swivel Seat, Crocodile 1, Candle 1
Tuesday	Mars	Muscles and male reproductive organs	Marching in Place, Side Stretch, Stretch, Chair, Dog, Paddle Boat, Bridge
Wednesday	Mercury	Brain and nervous system	Crossover, Standing Cross, Chest Mover, Crawl, Little Cat, Rabbit, Quiet Frog,
Thursday	Jupiter	Digestive system	Hop, Stomach Inversion, Belly and Stomach Stretch, Leaf, Side Stretches and Knee Stand, Crocodile 2, Candle 2
Friday	Venus	Balance and female reproductive organs, kidneys, adrenal system	Loose Arm Swing, Pendulum, Pyramid, Side Balance, Grasshopper, Cobra, Turtle
Saturday	Saturn	Bones, joints, and metabolism	Plucking Stars, Bird in the Nest, Arm Bends and Stretches, Arm Circles, Leg Circles, Candle 3, Little Bear

INDEX OF YOGA POSES

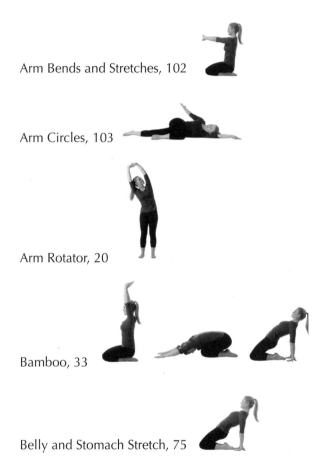

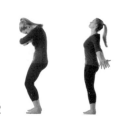

Blade, 22

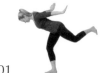

Bird in the Nest, 101

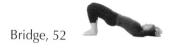

Bridge, 52

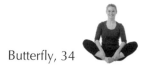

Broth Mixer, 36

Butterfly, 34

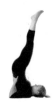

Chest Expander, 25

Chest Mover, 61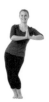

Chest Twist, 21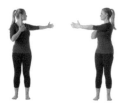

Closing Resting Position, 26 [*ff*]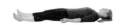

Cobra, 92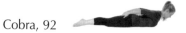

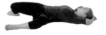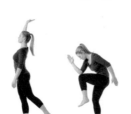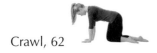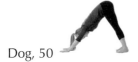

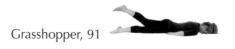
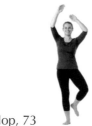 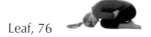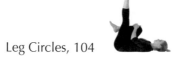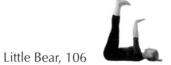

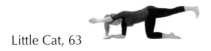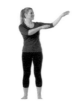

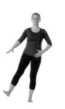

Pendulum, 88

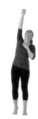

Plucking Stars, 100

Pyramid, 89

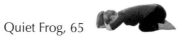

Quiet Frog, 65

Rabbit, 64

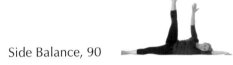

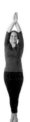

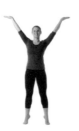

St. Andrew's Cross, 24

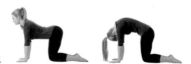

Stomach Inversion, 74

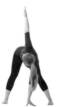

Stretch, 48

Swivel Seat, 37

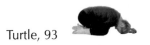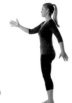

ABOUT THE AUTHOR

Gertrud Hirschi has been director of her yoga school in Zurich since 1982, where she teaches yoga in accordance with the latest medical findings. She frequently holds seminars and lectures, and has been a guest lecturer in managerial courses at the World Economic Forum in Davos, Switzerland. She is the author of many books on the subjects of yoga, mudras, and mantras, which have been translated into over eighteen languages. She is the author of *Basic Yoga for Everybody,* and *Mudras: Yoga in Your Hands*.

TO OUR READERS

Conari Press, an imprint of Red Wheel/Weiser, publishes books on topics ranging from spirituality, personal growth, and relationships to women's issues, parenting, and social issues. Our mission is to publish quality books that will make a difference in people's lives—how we feel about ourselves and how we relate to one another. We value integrity, compassion, and receptivity, both in the books we publish and in the way we do business.

Our readers are our most important resource, and we appreciate your input, suggestions, and ideas about what you would like to see published.

Visit our website at *www.redwheelweiser.com* to learn about our upcoming books and free downloads, and be sure to go to *www.redwheelweiser.com/newsletter* to sign up for newsletters and exclusive offers.

You can also contact us at *info@rwwbooks.com*.

Conari Press
an imprint of Red Wheel/Weiser, LLC
65 Parker Street, Suite 7
Newburyport, MA 01950
www.redwheelweiser.com